# A Message of Hope

## FROM A 24 YEAR CANCER SURVIVOR

### A PHENOMENAL STORY OF
### FAITH, HOPE, LOVE & COURAGE

BY

# PATRICIA A. PENN PIERRE

CONTACT INFORMATION

Author

Tricia.Pierre@yahoo.com

Co- Author

melvin.pierre@yahoo.com

Editing provided by:

m_letha@bellsouth.net

# Introduction

As you read this book, I'd like to make one thing clear from the very beginning. This book is not an attempt to **convince you** of anything or **convert you** to anything. Nor is it an attempt to **persuade you** to **believe anything** that **I believe** or to join any religious organization, operation or affiliation. It is **A Message of Hope** for those who may have experienced or may be experiencing the same type of challenges that I did. It's **A Message of Hope** for you and every member of your family...... because, if your family is like my family, when I was diagnosed with breast cancer, it affected every member of my family in one way or the other. Some were able to express their feelings and some were not able to express their feelings. But they all surrounded me with their love and support ...and for that, I am truly grateful.

As we all know, every diagnosis of cancer is unique and there are certainly no guarantees. I'm a **living witness** that a diagnosis of cancer is not the end of the world. On the contrary, it was the beginning of a whole new world... with a new meaning and a new purpose. My mother, my husband, my family and many of my friends have suggested, over the years, that I should write a book about my experience because...as they all said.... "**somebody** needs to hear your story." If you are that "**somebody**," this message is for **you**. I'm talking directly to **you!** So I invite you to join me and "step back in time" as I share what some would see as a tragedy....but one that I see as a triumph.

This is a true story...a story of **Faith, Hope, Love & Courage.** In 1987, I was diagnosed with breast cancer. Within a 90 day period, I had a double mastectomy and found myself **breasts-less**. This was one of the most challenging times in my life. By no means am I trying to tell <u>you</u> what to do or even suggest what you should do ... if you ever have to face a situation like this. Please don't get the impression that I'm trying to force my beliefs, opinions, values, testimony or experiences on you.

My goal is simply to encourage you to keep your head "to the sky" (from whence cometh your help) and to continue moving forward **with great expectations.** I want to share with you, what **I** did...step by step...during my time of turmoil. Feel free to use **all** of it....**parts** of it....or **none** of it. That's up to you.

If you or any of your family members have ever had to face cancer...or may ever have to face cancer, at some point in the future, this book was written especially for **YOU.** I have been through what you may be going through or may have to go through. So I understand your fears, your apprehensions, your challenges, your pain and your suffering. If I can give hope to just **one** person in this universe, then writing this book and sharing my experience and testimony is well worth it.

Please know that you are not alone.

# This Book Is Dedicated To

<u>My Dad</u>

Samuel Penn, Sr.

<u>My Mom</u>

Beatrice Scott Penn

**My Sisters & Brothers**

Frances

Catherine

Samuel

Benny

Elaine

Julia

**My Husband, Son & Grandson**

Melvin, Sr.

Melvin, Jr.

Melvin Pierre, III

**<u>My Extended Family & Friends:</u>** Dr. Tanyanika Phillips, Anthony Penn, Kenneth & Charmaine Penn Johnson, Jim Nasser, Zemedah L. Watlington, Barbara Penn, Ruth Penn, Leon Miller, Sr., Leon Miller, Jr., Robert Scott, Edward & Louise Scott, Harriet White, The Late Harold White, Ethel Williams, Karl Fields, Bob & Carol Clemens, Sarah & Jessie Cainion, Pamela Fisher, Deshan Marlow, Charles Smith, Brenda Hogan, Joyce Clark, Theorlyn Rayborn, Pastor Deidre Carter, Adrian & Yolanda Curtis, Michelle Jones, Joycelyn Smith, Curtis & Courtney Wright, Marion Williams, Robert & Geraldine Preston, Debra Austin,  Noreen Workman, April Richard, Linda & Nina Swanson, Ruth, Karen & Kislyck Halsey, Brian & Cheryl Banks, The Parker & Peggy Perret Family, The Bruce & Myra Carter Family. Clyde & Pat Bond, Sonya Davis, Sean Williams, John Jansen, Charles Terry, Josie Gilbert, Jacqueline McChristian, Jane Tureaud, Jeffrey Penn & Tyrone Penn, Oliver and Wanda Bell, Johnny & Betty Vickers, Sr., Joseph & Betty Roberson, Pastor Kenneth Samuel, The Deacon Board and The Victory Congregation and all my other friends and prayer partners who are too numerous to mention. Your prayers were answered!!!

**<u>THANKS</u>** for your friendship and for all of your prayers, encouragement, love, and support over the years. There will always be a special place in my heart for you.

I Love You All

# Special Thanks

We are living examples of God's love and witnesses to His Glory and as such we would be remiss without giving thanks to those who served as instruments in the divine plan for our family.

In phase 1 of God's plan, we express our sincerest appreciation to Doctors Meyer Kaplan, Salvador Caputto, William Leon, and John Church. We thank the clinical breast cancer team and all those who helped in medical oncology including pathologists, radiologists, pharmacists, nurses, technicians, and administrators at Touro Infirmary Hospital, New Orleans Louisiana.

In phase 2 of God's divine plan, for dedication to the field of oncology and compassionate care of patients with cancer we acknowledge our niece.

Dr. Tanyanika Phillips

and so many others for their tireless efforts including:

Dr. Nithya Palanisamy

Dr. David Gerber

Dr. Harris Naina

Dr. Jad Wakim

Dr. Anderson, Dr. Flippo, Dr. Cardinal

The medical staff and administrative staff at Texas Presbyterian Allen

The entire medical staff and administrative staff at UT Southwestern Medical Center Zale- Lipshy and Parkland Hospitals.

All Adult and Children Hospitals, Organizations, Research, Resource and Support Centers whose mission is to find a cure and eliminate cancer as a major health problem by preventing cancer, saving lives and diminishing suffering from cancer, through research, education, advocacy and service.

# You **Are** Making A Difference

# THANKS FOR ALL YOU DO!!!

As God prepares us for the next phase of our journey, we will continue to stand on Faith, Hope, Love & Courage.

# Table of Contents

# It Started With A Cough In 1987

I had just celebrated my 40th birthday in May, 1987. It was a beautiful summer that year and was coming to an end. But a storm was brewing that would change the entire course and focus of my life. It started with a normal cough and progressed into a persistent cough.....and continued to the point where I became hoarse and lost my voice.

A chest x-ray, in July, 1987, revealed nodules in my left breast and suggested that nodules may be present in my right breast as well. I was hoping and praying that they were benign fibroid tumors since I had a history of developing those types of tumors. We were making big plans for one of my favorite months..... August...because my momma, who was born on August 22nd, was about to celebrate her 73rd birthday. And my son, who was born on August 15th, was about to celebrate his 19th birthday.

In addition to celebrating all of the birthdays, I always looked forward to the month of August because that was the month we got new clothes and made preparations to go back to school (which I really enjoyed ). But this August, in 1987, in my 40th year, life would be very different from the other 39. This would be the beginning of one of the most challenges phases of my life.

<u>08-05-87</u>   A biopsy revealed carcinoma of both breasts

I must have been under some form of anesthesia......but I do remember waking up, after the biopsy procedure, and looking up and being surrounded by a room full of family members who were all crying big tears. My room and the waiting room were overflowing with my family members. They came from everywhere........from all parts of the city. The nurse said "You are truly loved. All of your family is here for you." Looking at the concerned looks on their faces and all of the tears, I got the impression they thought I was about to die. My doctors asked everybody to leave my room except my mother and my husband. And I clearly remember four words that kept ringing in my ears:

# You Have Breast Cancer!!!

Get A Cancer Screening Today

At that point, I was in a complete state of shock and disbelief. I have Breast Cancer??? Me??? Breast Cancer??? That can't be true. Not me!

Can you imagine being blind-sided and flattened by a Mack truck traveling at 100mph? Can you imagine losing all the wind out of your sails….all the joy in your heart…….and all the "life" in your spirit and feeling like your body has been transformed from a **solid** form to a silhouette of a body in an instant? That will give you an idea of the impact those four words had on me that day.

I didn't know **what to expect**….but I knew, instinctively, **who to call on.**

I started to cry out softly…

**Oh**

**My**

**GOD!**

And I cried out again…a little louder….

# Oh

# My

# GOD!!

And I cried out again…a little bit louder….

# Oh
# My
# GOD!!!

And I cried out again…louder than before……

# Oh
# My
# GOD!!!!

And I cried out again…as loud as I possibly could…..

# Oh
# My
# GOD!!!!!

**The more I cried out, the more I could feel my spirit getting stronger and stronger**

Then Momma whispered these words in my ear…with tears in both eyes……

"Don't cry baby. It's gonna be all right. God is not finished with you yet. He's got a lot more left for you to do. I love you so much. And I'm going to be here to take care of you."

Now It Was

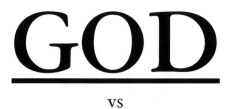

GOD

vs

Breast Cancer

And the breast cancer didn't seem so big anymore.....

The more I cried out to God, the smaller my challenge became... because I knew that He was the **one and only one** who could fix this. I'm talking about the God who created heaven and earth... the sun...the moon... the stars and all the life in the universe. The Timekeeper who controls night and day and every breath <u>we</u> take.....and how long we can stay. The One who created the rivers, the streams, the oceans, sharks, whales and all the other fish in the sea... the forest, the wildlife, the hills and valleys.... the One who planted the trees and vegetation on top of mountains that man has yet to see. I'm talking about the God who created Adam and Eve.....and you and me....and every single cell in our body. The One who was there in the beginning and will be there in the end. That's the One I'm talking about.

It was very clear to me: The One who created my body is the One who would heal my body. I came to the realization that God had the **solution** long before I even had this problem. To those of you who are reading this book, I'd like to say that whatever you may be going through, at this point in your life, whether it's related to cancer or any other challenge, I would encourage you to focus on The Problem Solver and not the problem! Focusing on the "**Problem Solver** as opposed to focusing on the **problem**" is an excerpt from a sermon by Dr.Kenneth L.Samuel at Victory Church in Stone Mountain, GA. And it's so true... because If I had focused on the problem, I would have missed out on the opportunity to interact with the Problem Solver and witness His Power as he interceded on my behalf.

As I look back on this series of events, that persistent cough and the hoarseness were like receiving **G-MAIL** from God. The cough was a "message in disguise" and HIS message was very clear:

## You Have Mail

*"Patricia.......take action now and get to the doctor......
because you and I are going to work together to solve this problem.
Please know...in advance....in your heart, mind, body, soul
and spirit...that I will be with you every step of the way."*

### End of Message

(The <u>G-Mail</u> I'm Talking About Has Nothing To Do With
G-Mail Accounts On The Internet)

**I BELIEVE** all of us are directly **connected** to our creator and, long before anybody ever knew how to spell the word "computer," God had already created the greatest central processing unit ( CPU ) that has ever been or ever will be created......the **human brain.** If we listen very carefully, we can "hear" the G-MAIL He personally sends to our **INBOX.** I found out you don't need a high-speed internet connection to hear or read HIS mail. Turn off everything and just meditate in a quiet place and listen. And you will hear his **VOICE-ACTIVATED G-MAIL.** I am so thankful He took the time to send me a "message through a cough" and the hoarseness that forced me to see the doctor. I'm so glad I was not too busy to hear, read and understand His mail because that message saved my life!!!

At any rate, after my diagnosis and after exploring all of the options that were available to me at that time, I knew one thing for sure:

No matter what I was about to face, I knew, from the very beginning, I could count on God and His Word. As I look back over 64 years of living, 1987 was the **<u>"defining moment"</u>** when God and His Word came "alive" in my life. Cancer was too big for me or any other human being to solve and face alone. But I knew, beyond a shadow of a doubt, that the Creator of my body was the **One and only One** who had the power to heal the body He created. He did not have to wait to find a cure for cancer because He had the solution to my cancer long before I had the problem!!! I am truly grateful to all of the doctors, scientists, researchers and organizations, around the world, who have dedicated their lives, missions and resources to finding the cure to this dreaded disease......but I knew then....and I know now, beyond a shadow of a doubt, that God already has the answers to all of the questions and the solutions to all of the problems. That's the **FIRST THING** I knew and He's the One I called on **FIRST**. For every action, there's a reaction. Calling on Him **FIRST** formed the very foundation for my recovery.

I invited Him in and asked Him to take charge of the situation......and take charge He did!!! He came to my house in New Orleans, Louisiana and alerted me that I needed to go to the doctor's office for the check-up that, ultimately, revealed the problem. He was in the Operating Room, the Recovery Room, the Chemotherapy Sessions, the Doctors Offices and all of the other places you would want and need Him to be. He walked with me and He talked with me every step of the way....and He made sure I knew He was there!!! I found out, for myself, that when you put God in the ring with cancer or any other problem, that's like a fixed fight. I had complete and unwavering, child-like **FAITH** that my outcome would be favorable. And it was!!!

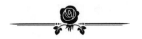

# Early Detection Will Increase Your Chances For Survival

__Early Detection__ played a very big part in my case and could play a very big part in your case as well. __Consult your doctors for your medical advice.__

Early __detection__ and the __actions__ you take **after that** can make the difference. Here's a true and painful story: After I was diagnosed with breast cancer, one of my best girl friends did a self-examination and discovered an area on her breast that just didn't feel right. But she was afraid to go to the doctor to find out what it was. She waited and waited and waited...and when she finally went to the doctor, it was too late because the cancer had spread. Instead of us having an opportunity to continue our beautiful friendship, I had to attend her funeral. That was so hard to deal with. So we have to be vigilant and do **our** part if we want God to do **His** part.

God says

# IF YOU WILL.......I WILL.

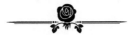

<u>Do Your Part.......Get A Cancer Screening Today</u>

# *Take Action Now!!!*

Make sure you have all of your examinations done on a regular basis and encourage everybody in your family and all of your friends to do the same.

# **YOU** CAN MAKE A DIFFERENCE in somebody's life:

Call a minimum of 10 of your family members, friends and associates. If they are females, encourage them to get a (1) mammogram (2) PAP Smear (3) colonoscopy and (4) a complete physical. If they are male friends, encourage them to get a (1) Prostate Check Up (2) complete physical (3) Colonoscopy and any other exams that are recommended by their doctors.

Remember the number 10. You mission is to encourage a **MINIMUM of 10** family members, friends and associates.........
and then to encourage them to encourage others.

| | |
|---|---|
| 10 encouraging 10 = | 100 |
| 100 encouraging 10 = | 1,000 |
| 1000 encouraging 10 = | 10,000 |
| 10000 encouraging 10 = | 100,000 |
| 100000 encouraging 10 = | 1,000,000 |

This heightened awareness and early detection will cause lives to be saved.

## YOU CAN MAKE A DIFFERENCE

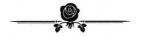

# If Cancer is Detected, Take Swift and Aggressive Action

If cancer is detected anywhere in your body, you and your doctors have to be more aggressive than the cancer. You have to declare war on this cancer immediately. This is not the time for a "pity party." It's not the time for the "why me Lord" conversation. It's time to (1) locate (2) isolate (3) terminate and (3) eliminate any and all opportunities for that cancer to continue its path of destruction. If you want to have an "opportunity" to live, **whatever has to go**...... **has to go**!!! I don't want anything on me that can destroy the rest of me. It's that simple.

Another friend of mine was diagnosed with breast cancer and stated, emphatically, that no doctor was going to cut on her and remove her breasts. She was under the "false impression" that she was going to continue living life as she had been.... without taking any actions to deal with the diagnosis. It's my understanding that, at the time of her diagnosis, she was pregnant with twins. Needless to say, we went to a funeral for three. She and her unborn children were all buried together. One of those children may have grown up to become the doctor who would discover the cure for cancer. But they never got an opportunity to live!

That funeral made a lasting impression on my husband. When I was diagnosed with breast cancer and tried to feel sorry for myself....worrying about how my husband would feel looking at me everyday with no breasts, he made a statement that I'll never forget:

"I'd rather have you with **no breasts** then to have to bury you with two breasts sticking up looking at me!!!!! What do we need breasts for anyway???" (MP)

Our marriage was far from perfect.... but all of my worries about how he would feel about breasts or no breasts and hair or no hair were unfounded because this is the **single event** that brought us closer together as husband and wife. This is the event that changed both of our lives for the better. In January, 2011, we celebrated 43 years of marriage.

So we, as a couple, were finally on the same page and took very aggressive actions during our time of turmoil and were very eager to locate, isolate, terminate and eliminate any parts that needed to be eliminated in order for us to continue.

I was always taught that God will help those who help themselves. If you have any type of cancer in your body but are not willing to take the proper and prudent steps to help yourself increase your chances of survival, you may find yourself in a position where you'll be meeting God a little sooner than you anticipated.

If it'll make you feel better, get a 2<sup>nd</sup> opinion or a 3<sup>rd</sup> opinion to confirm the diagnosis.......and then take **immediate and aggressive action** to stop the cancer before it has an opportunity to create additional cancer cells and stop you!

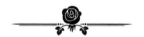

# You Have Breast Cancer! — Now What?

**First Things First:** The very first thing I decided to do was to move from the driver's seat >>>>to the passenger seat and ask God to take over the driver's seat because we were about to travel down a rough and dangerous road that I had never seen. It made no sense to me to stay behind the wheel and ask God if He wanted to go along for the ride as a passenger in my vehicle. On the contrary, I wanted to be a passenger in His vehicle. I knew that I had to surrender completely.....and I did. I also knew I could stand on his Word....and I did.

"Trust in the LORD with all thine heart; and lean not unto thine own understanding. In all thy ways acknowledge him, and he shall direct thy paths." (Proverbs 3:5-6)

I had **no** understanding about breast cancer. So I could not lean on my understanding. I put all of my trust in the Lord. I acknowledged Him and He did exactly what He said He would do. He directed my path.

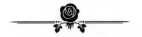

# The Power of Serenity, Faith, Hope, Love & Courage

I had to get ready for the fight of my life. One thing I understood, from the very beginning, is **WHO** was and still is in control. All of my doctors were highly recommended specialists in their fields. While I had confidence in my doctors' abilities to do what they were trained to do, I had complete **FAITH** in God, the Creator, because He is the One who **made** every single cell in my body and He is the only One who has the power to **heal** every cell in my body........and He would be the One guiding my doctors' hands, minds and instruments to remove every malignant cell that needed to be removed. This is the time in my life when my faith increased to a level I had never experienced.

In addition to **FAITH**, I knew I also needed **SERENITY**. Each and every day of my life, I ask God for the **SERENITY** to accept the things I cannot change. There was no way I could change the fact that I had just been diagnosed with breast cancer. I always ask for the **COURAGE** to change the things I can. So I asked Him to give me the **COURAGE** to made the right decisions, take the right actions and face any and all challenges that I was about to face. And the **WISDOM** to know the difference. What difference? The difference between those things I **cannot** change and the things I **can** change. Oftentimes, we go through life worrying about things we **cannot possibly** change and lose focus on the things we **can** change. That's why we need the **WISDOM** to know the difference.

God, grant me the serenity

To accept the things I cannot change;

Courage to change the things I can;

And wisdom to know the difference.

# The Penn Family
# All For One......And One For All

We were always taught that whenever any one of us had a problem, a challenge, or whatever, the rest of us would come together, as a team, to help resolve that problem or challenge. If any one of us got "knocked down," for any reason, everybody else in the family would spring into action to lift that person back up. That's the way it's always been in the Penn Family and that's the way it is to this day. So when I was "knocked down," they all made sure that I was not "knocked out." They all came together and surrounded me with the **LOVE** and **SUPPORT** I needed to make it through.  My momma moved in to my home and stayed until she knew, for sure, that I could take care of myself and my family once again. She was 73 years old at that time and was still very active in everything she wanted to do. She did whatever needed to be done....cooking, cleaning, crying, praying, encouraging, and nurturing me back to health. She took care of my house and her house simultaneously. She made sure everything in **my** household would still run smoothly. We never missed a beat. Her love and support kept me in a positive frame of mind and gave me the strength and the determination to keep moving forward, with great expectations. That same love and support kept my husband in a position to continue running his insurance agency and to be available to take me to the hospital, the doctors, the chemotherapy sessions and everything else in between.

Momma loved all of her children, unconditionally, and whenever any of us needed her support, she was always there.

In the final analysis, she took care of all seven of us more than we ever had to take care of her. We celebrated her 95th birthday on August 22, 2009. She went home to be with the Lord on December 24, 2009. I was blessed to have the opportunity to be by her side on the last night of her life (12-23-09). As we said our goodbyes that night, my final words to her were "I Love You" and her final words to me were "I Love You More." I was truly blessed to have her as my mom. I could not have asked for a better mom. Not only was she my mom........she was my very best friend and I miss her dearly.

As for my household, thirty-six (36) months prior to my diagnosis, my husband had started his own insurance agency on August 15, 1984 and it was growing at a very rapid pace. Business was brisk. The phone was ringing "off the hook." He was working until 10pm. almost every day of the week. However, when I needed his **LOVE** and **SUPPORT,** during my time of trouble, in 1987, he was right there, by my side, everyday and every night and continued to run the insurance agency without ever letting any of his clients or associates know what he was going through.

We had what we thought was a very good medical plan but I also remember that we had to pay over $33,000 of out of pocket expenses to supplement what the insurance company paid. The "financial side" of the battle was a tremendous burden that created an almost unbearable level of stress. In addition to the $400 per month for the medical insurance premiums, now we had to make arrangements to pay off the $33,000 of unpaid medical bills. While we were doing our best to stay current on all of these new obligations (in addition to our regular household expenses), the health insurance company started increasing the monthly insurance premiums in an effort to "force" us out so they could be "off the hook." Upon renewal, the $400 per month was increased to $600 per month. When the policy was renewed again, the monthly payment increased to $900 per month….then $1,200 per month….then $1,400 per month… then $1,800 per month until we couldn't take it no more.

After having his own agency, in New Orleans, for 15 years, my husband decided to sell the insurance agency and relocate to Atlanta to work with one of his best managers ever….who also happens to be one of the nicest human beings on this planet. Needless to say, the compensation package included health insurance to protect our family. With cancer as a pre-existing condition, we knew it would be virtually impossible to secure affordable health insurance on our own. It's amazing how God works through other people to make a way out of (what appears to us to be) "no way." God chose to work this situation out through my husband's favorite manager who had no idea what we were going through. We were "touched by an angel" named **Bob Clemens.** Years later, we shared that story with him and his wife and thanked him again for the role he played in our lives at a very crucial time. We will be friends until the end of time!!! When that assignment was over in Atlanta and it was time to move on, God worked through two other angels to help us make a smooth transition from Atlanta to Gonzales, Louisiana. We were covered on both ends by **Courtney Wright** in Atlanta and **John Jansen** in Louisiana. One made sure we had a "smooth take-off" and the other made sure we had a "safe landing."

In the summer of 1963, our lives were "touched by an angel" named **Marion Williams** (my husband's Aunt). My husband is not the type of person who likes to go to dances or events of that nature. However, in 1963, when he was 15 years old, his Aunt

Marion "literally" forced him to go to his first dance. I remember him asking me five words when I met him at that dance: "May I have this dance?" And that's how we met. We were married in January, 1968 and celebrated 43 years of marriage on January 13, 2011. As a result of our marriage, we have one son, Melvin Pierre, Jr. and one grandson, Melvin Pierre, III. God worked through his Aunt Marion to put Melvin, Sr. in the exact spot where he needed to be on that particular night...... because that's the **one and only time** I would have had an opportunity to meet him. In my opinion, that was a part of God's plan for our lives. What would have happened had he not listened to his Aunt on that night? That's a scary thought.

At any rate, in August, 1987, we had been married for 19 years and had not had the best marriage in the world. But the cancer diagnosis and our need to pull together to work through this challenge is the event that "solidified" our marriage and our commitment to one another. We became closer than ever. We became best friends. Finally, we became ONE.

So in the final analysis, I was ready for the battle that I was faced with.... because I had all I needed to overcome this "challenge."

(1) **COMPLETE and UNWAVERING CHILD-LIKE FAITH IN GOD.**

(2) **SERENITY & PEACE IN MY SPIRIT.**

(3) **AN "ANGELIC" TEAM of DOCTORS & SPECIALISTS.**

(4) **SURROUNDED BY THE LOVE & ENCOURAGEMENT OF MY FAMILY.**

(5) **COURAGE** to make the right decisions and take the right actions.

(6) **HOPE** that everything would work in my favor….**AND IT DID!!!**

So here's a message for you: No matter what you might be going through in your life right now, never lose **HOPE**…..because it ain't over until God says it's over. If He wants it to be over….and want you to come back home…..then it'll be over… on "this side"….with a new beginning on the "other side." If that's the case, you'll be absent from the body….but you'll be in the presence of the Lord (if you live your life according to His Word). And that's the ultimate goal anyway!!!

You probably know somebody who heard a doctor say "I've done all that I can do….and all that I know how to do." And then God stepped in and said "I'll Do The Rest!!!…..I'll Take It From Here!!!" And that person may still be with us today. So Never…Never…Never… Lose **HOPE**. When you lose **HOPE**, you've lost it all.

# It Ain't Over Until GOD Says It's Over!

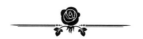

# I Was Blessed With An "Angelic" Team of Doctors

God is the **SOURCE** and He works through the **RESOURCES** (in my case......the doctors and their skill sets). They do what they've been trained to do and He does the rest. While the doctors have been trained to do the analyses, diagnoses, administer the drugs that are necessary to fight this dreaded disease, perform the required surgical procedures and the sutures that are necessary to reunite the edges of the cut or wound, it is God who has to mend it back together and bring forth the healing. It's a beautiful thing to watch the "physical" side and the "spiritual" side working together on our behalf. I'll share some of those experiences with you as we move forward.

In my case, I was blessed to be surrounded with an "angelic team of doctors." Doctor Meyer Kaplan made the initial diagnosis. Dr. Kaplan introduced me to Dr. William Leon, who performed my surgeries. They both highly recommended Dr. Salvador Caputto, my Oncologist, and Dr. John Church, was my Plastic Surgeon. What an awesome team of doctors!!!

Here's a recap of one of the most challenging times in my life as recorded in the doctor's report:

## 08-13-87

| | |
|---|---|
| Preoperative Diagnosis: | Carcinoma of the left breast and probably the right breast |
| Postoperative Diagnosis: | Carcinoma of both breasts. |
| Name of Operation: | Left Modified Radical Mastectomy |
| Surgeon: | Dr. William Leon |

I'm sharing all of this information with you because **somebody….somewhere…in some country** is in this same situation right now...and may be looking at a report just like this one. I want to encourage you to keep your head to the sky and not on the ground. Just because you hear the word cancer or carcinoma don't necessarily mean your world is about to come to an end.

## *One of my favorite passages in the Bible is the 23rd Psalm:*

1. The LORD is my shepherd; I shall not want.

2. He maketh me to lie down in green pastures; he leadeth me beside the still waters.

3. He restoreth my soul; he leadeth me in the paths of righteousness for his name's sake.

4. Yea, though I walk through the valley of the shadow of death, I will fear no evil; for thou art with me; thy rod and thy staff they comfort me.

5. Thou preparest a table before me in the presence of mine enemies; thou anointest my head with oil; my cup runneth over.

6. Surely goodness and mercy shall follow me all the days of my life; and I will dwell in the House of the LORD forever.

### *Here is one of the reasons why I was not afraid......*

Yea, though I walk through the valley of the shadow of death, I will fear no evil; for thou art with me; thy rod and thy staff they comfort me.

As you continue to read my testimony, you will know that everything in the 23rd Psalm has been activated in my life. And since God is no respecter of person, the promises in this 23rd Psalm can be activated in your life as well.

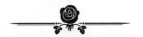

# A Miracle in The Operating Room

Over the years, I've had several surgeries, for a variety of ailments, but never had an experience like the one I had with Dr. William Leon, my main surgeon. As we entered the operating room for this radical mastectomy, Dr. Leon asked for permission to pray:

"Mrs. Pierre…would it be O.K. with you if we prayed before the surgery?"

WOW!!! That put a smile on my face, tears in my eyes and joy in my spirit. It was a confirmation that God was going to be the "Chief Surgeon" in the operating room and Dr. Leon was going to be His Assistant. God was going to work through the hands, heart and mind of my surgeon. When Doctor Leon knelt down at the head of the gurney to pray, he humbled himself before God and put me and my situation in the hands of God. What a comforting feeling!!! After the prayer, I drifted off into "la la land" and didn't feel anything that happened during my procedure.

Now that's what I'm talking about when I say it's a beautiful thing to watch the "physical" side and the "spiritual" side working together on your behalf.

Just like any other human being would react, when I first heard the diagnosis of breast cancer, I was in total shock and disbelief. I was broken down to my very core. My heart, mind, body, soul, spirit and confidence needed restoration.

And once again, I took refuge and found comfort in the 23rd Psalm:

3. He <u>restoreth </u>my soul; he leadeth me in the paths of righteousness for his name's sake.

4. Yea, though I walk through the valley of the shadow of death,

# I will fear no evil; 

for **thou** <u>art with me</u>; thy rod
and thy staff <u>they comfort me.</u>

That experience, in the operating room, is one that I cherish to this very day and will never forget. It was truly a **miracle** in the operating room.

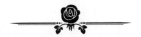

# Where Did My Breast Go?

After the diagnosis of breast cancer, I knew if I wanted to have an "opportunity" to **live**, my breasts would have to be removed. There was no question about that. I understood that very clearly. However, after the surgery, as the anesthesia was wearing off, I kept feeling for my left breast and I kept asking my momma and my husband where it was. Reality started to set in. Where did my breast go? What did they do with it? What did they do with it? It had been a part of me for so many years. Could I touch it one more time? Could I see it again….one more time? I wanted to see the inside of it so I could have a better understanding of what had actually happened to my breast. What is carcinoma? I wanted my doctor to show me what it looked like on the inside of my breast. I wanted him to explain it to me in plain English. I wanted to know. I cried and cried and cried. Most females can relate to that feeling.

On the other hand, I am grateful this carcinoma had been discovered **early** enough to save my life and had not had an opportunity to spread all over my body. August, 2011 is a milestone in my life and marks the 24th year of my recovery.

That's a direct gift from God of 8,760 days. When I look back over my 64 years of life (23,360 days), God has blessed me and my family so much that **I can't tell it all.** As the saying goes....if He don't do another thing in my life, He's already done enough!!!!

# I Am Truly Grateful

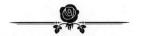

# After The Operation, I Had Another Mind-Boggling Experience

By the time I regained consciousness, I was in my room. I had no pain in the area where my left breast use to be….but the pain in my left arm was excruciating. It felt like my left arm had been broken into pieces. I found out later that some of the lymph nodes under my left arm pit had to be removed and that was the source of this pain. So I asked the nurse for some pain medication. The medication that I was given for pain caused me to hallucinate. I've never been on an LSD "trip" ……so I can't verify how that feels…. but whatever she gave me took me "around the world and back" on a journey somewhere that I've never been and don't ever want to go back to again. When I came back to my senses, I asked the nurse about the drug that I had been given and was told that it was morphine. That was the end of asking for pain medication!!!

The doctors were absolutely amazed that I was able to continue my recovery without that "powerful" pain medication. But I had a **"tried and tested solution"** for the pain. And I didn't need a prescription for that.

When the pain came back again, I started to **PRAY** and asked God to take away the pain that I was experiencing and to give me some peace so that I could sleep through the night. I prayed myself to sleep that night and had a very peaceful night of rest. The point I'm trying to make here is that God answers **PRAYERS.**

Within a few days of my surgery, I was sitting up in my bed and my chair and taking short walks as prescribed by my doctors. I was doing so well, physically and mentally, that my oncologist asked me to meet with one of his other patients and "have a talk" with her to cheer her up. Her surgery was very similar to one I had. We became the best of friends during our recovery. We even tried to schedule some of our chemotherapy sessions together to keep each other strong and in a positive frame of mind. From the outset, she did not seem to have a strong support system like I had. From our conversations, I could sense some of the turmoil that she was going through. As time went on, our friendship blossomed. We both decided to have breast reconstructive surgery. After the surgery, she shared with me that her husband was not pleased with the outcome and that she was under a tremendous amount of stress and strain from him because he wanted to know what happened to the "nipples" on the implants. I sincerely hope you have a partner who is concerned about **YOU, your recovery, your health and your overall chances for survival...** as opposed to the cosmetics.

Overcoming the challenges of cancer, radiation, chemotherapy and everything else that goes with it is hard enough as it is and when you don't have the support, peace, and love in your home and in your spirit, it's very difficult to overcome cancer plus all of those additional burdens. Needless to say, she didn't make it very long under all of that pressure.

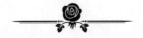

# Breast Reconstruction Because I Wanted To Feel Whole Again

In September, 1987, the second breast was removed. There was no need to wait and think about it. It had to be done. My husband and I agreed, in advance, that **whatever had to go.......had to go!!!** During the second operation, my breast reconstruction surgeon had joined the team. As soon as the right breast was removed, a breast implant was immediately inserted where the right breast had been. So when I woke up from that surgery, I felt much better because, at least, I had "something" in place that looked like a breast and would fit in a bra. The plan was to allow more time for the left breast area to heal and then place an implant in that area so I could feel "whole again." After the second implant had been installed, it was hard for anyone to tell what I had been through. They fit perfectly in a bra and I was "good to go." Unfortunately, the feeling of euphoria only lasted for a few months because one of the implants started leaking and we made a decision to have them both removed. Just like the original breasts, when I started to have problems with the implants, my husband was the first to say " they gotta go!!!" They were removed and that was the end of that. And we have not had the "implant conversation" for well over 22 years. I wanted to share this breast reconstruction story with you because there's somebody somewhere who is going through this very same scenario right now or may have already been through it. Fortunately, I was blessed with a husband who is concerned about **me** as opposed to cosmetics. At a time like this, it's all about **you**! Do what makes **you** feel good. Do what makes **you** feel better about the situation. Don't try to please others. You never will. This is not the time for that. This is **YOUR** Life.... It's **YOUR** Time. Enjoy the rest of **your** life.

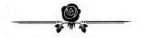

# A Miracle In The Midst Of Chemotherapy

So now it was time to face six months of chemotherapy. I had no idea what to expect or what effect those drugs would have on me. Here's what I "thought" I knew about chemotherapy: people who take chemotherapy lose their hair. It's amazing how things happen all around us, on a daily basis, but we never pay any attention to them... until we have to go through them for ourselves or with one of our loved ones. Prior to the first session, my husband and I joined hands, hearts, souls and prayed that Dr. Caputto, my oncologist, would mix "something" in with the chemotherapy drugs that would prevent me from losing my hair. Some folks are blessed with the ability to quote scriptures and verses in every book of the Bible. That's not us. We are not biblical scholars, bible experts and or anything like that. And it's good to know that we don't have to be. But we do know how to find what we need... when we need it. And we have complete Faith in God and His Word. We know that God **will do** what He **says** He **will do**. We all have the ability to "activate" His promises. So we started our prayer with the following passage in our hearts:

<u>Matthew 18:20 says, "For where two or three are gathered in my name, there I am among them."</u>

That's pretty straight forward. So this was our prayer: "**LORD**.....**YOU SAID**....that for where two or three are gathered in **your** name, there **you** would be among them." So we come before YOU tonight and know that YOU are here among us... as YOU said YOU would be... and ask that YOU would touch our oncologist and cause him to add something "special" to the chemotherapy drugs so that I will not lose my hair. All these things we pray, in JESUS name. AMEN.

That was the exact prayer we prayed.
We **Asked** and **HE Answered.**

## HE DELIVERED ONCE AGAIN!!!

During my first two chemotherapy sessions, I was a little nauseated and did whatever I could to settle my stomach. My husband escorted me to the first two sessions because we really didn't know what to expect or what was going to happen. I drove myself to all of the other sessions for the six months of chemotherapy and never had any other problems.

On top of all of that, I never lost my hair. The texture changed to the point where I did not have to have as many perms as I had in the past.....but once again, God had answered our prayer. My oncologist was even amazed that I did not lose my hair. I don't know if it's possible to add something "special" to chemotherapy drugs to help minimize hair loss....but, after the treatments, we told my oncologist about the prayer that we prayed before the sessions. So did Dr. Caputto add something "special" to the chemotherapy drugs or did God do it? We know one thing for a fact……..I didn't lose my hair and still have it to this day!!! God still answers prayers.

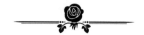

# Double Mastectomy, Reconstructive Surgery and a Hysterectomy!

In the six month period, from the initial diagnosis in August, 1987 to December, 1987, I had a Double Mastectomy, Reconstructive Surgery, Removal of the Implants. We were advised that the next area of attack could be the ovaries. So we made a swift and a conscious decision to have a Hysterectomy as well.  Our mind-set was **whatever has to go**...........has to go. Through it all, our faith grew stronger and stronger.  Never once did I ever entertain the "thought" that I was going to die.  I had so much more to do.

**Yea, though I walk through the valley
of the shadow of death,**

## I will  fear no evil;

**for thou art with me**; thy rod and thy
staff **they comfort me.**

I had to walk through the valley of the shadow of death......
but I feared no evil because God was with me.....just as He said

He would be. His rod and his staff comforted me throughout the entire process. I had no choice but to embrace the situation and the challenge and walk through it all by **FAITH** and not by sight.....because I had no sight. There was no way for me to **SEE** the results, in advance. Nobody in my family could tell me what was going to happen. I had to **Walk By Faith**.....and trust God and His Word. That, in itself, was very comforting because if you can't trust God, who can you trust? So I let go and let God have His way. There was no turning back! I was "all in." He was all I had.....and all I needed to have. I put it **all** in His hands!!! Everything was on the line. The life that he gave me was in His hands. I did my part....and stepped out on **Faith**....... and He did his part....... just like He said He would.

The message here is very clear: <u>**He will....if you will.**</u> We worked together, as a team, in order to bring about a recovery. This experience put me in a position to develop a "personal relationship" with God. While I was concerned about overcoming and recovering from cancer, He was concerned about my eternity. He was concerned about the "big picture." This is the event where he wrapped His arms around me and brought me through it all. And He made sure I knew it was Him and only Him. When God wants to do something "special" in your life, He does it in such a way that **you know** He was the **only one** who could have done it.

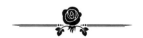

# I May Be Breasts-Less ...But I Am So Thank-Ful To Be Alive!!!

As we go through life, there are many choices we have to make. Where we are **TODAY** can be traced back to the choices we made **YESTERDAY**. I keep thinking about my friend who made the statement that "no doctor is going to cut on me and remove my breasts." So we buried her with both her breasts and both of her unborn children. On the other hand, I made a decision to eliminate whatever had to be eliminated so I could live to see another day. And here we are 24 years **after** that decision. I may be **Breasts-LESS**.....but I am so **Thank-FUL** to be here. **Life WITHOUT breasts** is so much better than **NO** life **WITH** breasts!!!

**I BELIEVE** we only have one life to live. So do whatever you need to do to continue living. Lose whatever you need to lose to keep on living. If you have to take chemotherapy and it causes you to lose you hair, lose it. You're still beautiful just as you are!!! Get a wig if that makes you feel better. You don't owe any explanation to anybody about anything! Don't worry about what other folks think or say about you. Do what YOU need to do to continue living. Impress yourself. In a situation like this, it's not about them, it's all about **YOU!!!**

As a matter of fact, many people who I "thought" were my friends ran away from me once they found out I had been diagnosed with cancer. Perhaps they were under the false impression they were going to "catch it" too. Or maybe they thought I was going to die. Many of them just disappeared. The calls stopped. The invitations stopped. It was as if I had developed leprosy or some other communicable disease.

Several of my "friends" developed cancer after I did and withdrew and went into a shell as if they were embarrassed or something. Whatever you do, don't let other people's opinions of you determine **your** opinion of you. As I said, at the beginning of this chapter, I may be **BREASTS-LESS** and have a flat chest nowadays…but I am so **THANKFUL** and **GRATEFUL** to be here 24 years after cancer. If this is what you are going through right now, hold your head up high because **you are not alone!!**

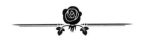

# Mrs. Pierre......You Are Cancer-Free!!!

At the end of all of the operations, scans, chemotherapy sessions, blood profiles and the battery of "check-point" tests, the **"moment of truth"** had arrived. It was time for the all-important summary consultation with my oncologist.

- How did I get breast cancer in the first place?

- What caused it?

- Where do I stand now?

- Did they get it all?

- What else do I need to do?

- What's the prognosis?

On the day of the consultation, Dr. Caputto, my oncologist, started the consultation with the following words: **Mrs. Pierre, I have some great news for you......You are Cancer-Free!!!!** I don't remember anything else after that...... but I do remember the following words......because, this time, the doctor's words were like music in my ears:

# Mrs. Pierre

# You

# are

# Cancer-Free!!!!

# Mrs. Pierre

# You

# are

# Cancer-Free!!!!

On the way home from that doctor's visit, we both had tears of joy in our eyes. And my husband shared this with me: a few nights before the appointment, he went into our bathroom at home...turned the lights out...and, in that darkness, had a "talk" with God and prayed a very special prayer (unbeknownst to me). In that prayer, he made a promise to God that if Dr. Caputto would say

### "Mrs. Pierre....You Are Cancer-Free"

he would officially join our church, get baptized and turn his life over to God. Dr. Caputto (on his own) had no way of knowing about the confirmation that my husband was seeking during that consultation.....but he started the consultation with the exact same words:

### "Mrs. Pierre....You Are Cancer-Free"

God answered that prayer through the words of our oncologist. It was a **direct confirmation.** And, as my husband promised during that very special prayer request, when the minister opened the doors of the church for membership at the next Sunday service, my husband was the first one to make it to the altar as a candidate for baptism. And, as he promised, he did, in fact, turn his life over to God and, as a result of that, we have been blessed so much, **we can't tell it all!!!!!!**

Twenty-four (24) years of check-up after check-up after check up after check-up have revealed the same results.....you are cancer-free.

# To **GOD** Be The Glory

Putting this book together has been a very emotional experience for me. It has taken me about six months to get to this point in the book. As I was proof reading it, I found myself "reliving" everything all over again. I had to do a triple-take when I read these words:

---

Twenty-four (24) years of check-up after check-up after check up after check-up have revealed the same results..... you are cancer-free.

# To **GOD** Be The Glory

---

By the time I got to this point, it was so emotional for me, I had to stop and take a break. But I kept thinking about the song, **Never Would Have Made It** ©. So I took a break, went to YOU TUBE © and watched **Dr. Marvin Sapp** (about two or three times) singing **Never Would Have Made It** ©. That song has a very special meaning to me. I "lost it" in the middle of that song........ because when I think about God's goodness and mercy and all of the things He has brought me and my family through in my 64 years....all I can say is **THANK YOU for your grace and mercy.** At first glance, the facts and the odds may have been stacked against me, but God turned everything around in my favor and brought me through. I never would have made it without Him.

# What an AWESOME GOD!!!

If you have access to a computer, I would encourage you to visit YOU TUBE © and watch the music video by **Dr. MARVIN SAPP** as he delivers this powerful message of thanks in **Never Would Have Made It** © 2008 Zomba Recording LLC. All of the versions are very good....but I prefer the "live" version at the following link:

http://www.youtube.com/watch?v=CklAwchIJ1A

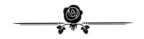

# My Family Is The Wind Beneath My Wings

I could never thank my family enough for all of the love, support and encouragement they provided me and continue to provide. It's a very comforting feeling to know that you are loved, unconditionally, by every member of your family and that you love each one of them, unconditionally, as well. But that's what we were taught. That's all we know.

I was blessed to have two of the best parents in the world.........and sisters and brothers who are inseparable, to this day. The "Penn Family" has always been a very happy and loving family. We are all in our 60s and 70s now.....but we're just as close, today, as we've always been. I'd like to take this opportunity to introduce you to "The Penn Family," and "The Pierre Family," starting with my Dad:

# My Dad,

# Samuel Penn, Sr.

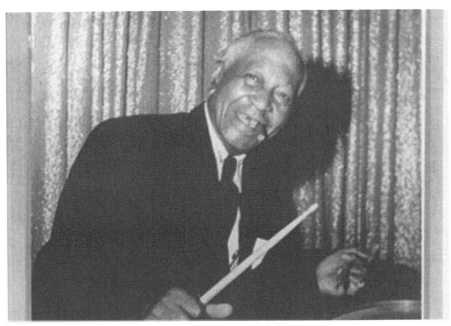

He was a well-known New Orleans Jazz Musician.....but, first and foremost, he was a wonderful human being and a wonderful father. His family meant the world to him. Dad..... Thank You so much for the life lessons you worked so hard to teach us. You led by example. You taught your boys how to be respectable men and how to provide strong foundations for their families. You worked hard and pampered your girls with everything that our little hearts desired. We learned so much about family values by watching the way you showered all of us with your love, laughter, support, guidance and dedication. God truly blessed us and smiled on us when he chose you to be the head of the Penn Family.

My dad was born on the 15<sup>th</sup> day of September, 1902 in Morgan City, Louisiana. From a young child, he was always interested in drums. His first drums were a tin tub, a cheese box and sticks made from chair rounds. In his early teens, he sat in with every band that went to Morgan City. In 1921, he came to New Orleans to work with the Chris Kelly Brass Band. By the time he moved to New Orleans, all of the New Orleans musicians already knew him. While in New Orleans, he met and married Beatrice Scott. As a result of that union, Frances, Catherine, Samuel, Jr., Benny, Letha-Elaine, Patricia and Julia were born. In the mid 50s, he took his own band, Penn and The Five Pennies, to Chicago. When he returned, he joined the World-Famous Preservation Hall Band. They traveled the world. He is featured on many of the recordings for The Kid Thomas Jazz Band as well as The Preservation Hall Band. He is best known as the drummer with The Kid Thomas Jazz Band and The Preservation Hall Band, with whom he played until his death on October 30, 1969 in LaGrange, Georgia. He was honored with a traditional New Orleans Jazz Funeral. Daddy......You are truly missed.

# My Mom

## Beatrice Scott Penn

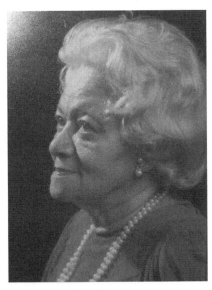

Momma was the "centerpiece" of our family. She was the one who set the "table of life" for us. She was our "Angel" right here on earth. We learned so much about life, love, faith, and family values by watching her in "action" on a daily basis. No matter what the problem was, she was always there to lift us up. She always knew what to say.....what to do.... and what needed to be done. We've always had (and continue to have) a very close-knit family. Each one of us talked to Momma at least three or four times a day...**everyday.** She was there **all** the time for **all** of us and we were there **all** the time for her. Whatever she wanted to do.....we were there. Wherever she wanted to go....we were there. Every Sunday, we would all meet up at "Grandma Bea's" house. She had a feast fit for a King & a Queen **every** Sunday.

She taught her boys how to stand up and be men and taught us girls how to be gracious ladies. She taught us how to love and respect ourselves and each other. If any of us even **"thought"** about going down the wrong path, she was there to make sure we stayed on the **right** path. **Wrong** was not an option in The Penn family. Talking negative about the Dallas Cowboys was also not an option. She loved football, baseball, basketball and golf (only when Tiger Woods played). She and my sister Frances, life-long Dallas Cowboys fans, were always ready for a "friendly battle" against the rest of us....most of whom are die-hard New Orleans Saints fans. What a wonderful and loving relationship we had with our mother! We had an incredible journey together and, for that, we are truly grateful.

She lived her life to the fullest until she was 95 years old. She took care of us more than we ever had to take care of her. She laughed until midnight on the very last night of her life. Before she went home to be with the LORD, on December 24, 2009, she made one final request and I quote **"no matter what happens, I want all of you to stay together."** She was truly one of a kind. Life will never be the same without her here with us. She was the love of our life. She was my best friend and will live in my heart **forever!**

My oldest sister, Frances, devoted her life to taking care of everything and anything that Momma and Daddy needed....... as well as the needs of her younger brothers and sisters. We all knew that Frances was **"in charge"** of the household when Momma and Daddy were at work (and she ran a **"tight** ship!") We couldn't "get over" on Momma.....nor could we "get over" on Frances. Momma taught her well. We are truly thankful for all she has done for all of us and, as of 2011, we still meet at "Grandma Bea and Frances" house on Sunday for the feast and our weekly reunion...... Frances is still **"our sister in charge"**......... and negative comments about the Dallas Cowboys are still not allowed!!!!!!!

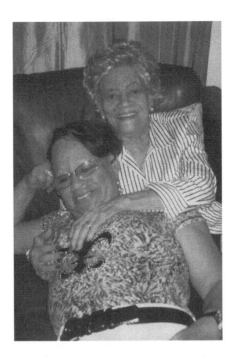

Me & My Momma on Her 95th and Final Birthday

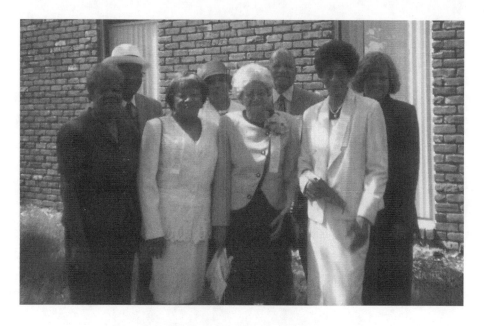

On Momma's 90th Birthday

My husband refers to my brothers and sisters as
"The Magnificent Seven."

## Introducing the Penn Family

2004

Catherine Williams

Benny Penn

Julia Fields

Letha-Elaine Miller

Momma

Samuel Penn, Jr.

Frances Penn

Patricia Pierre

# Introducing The Pierre Family

## Melvin Pierre, III- Melvin Pierre, Jr. - Patricia Pierre- Melvin Pierre, Sr.

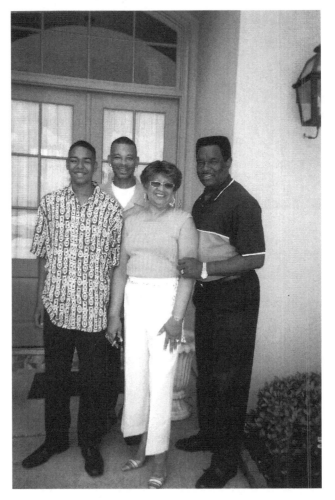

I met Melvin, Sr. in the summer of 1963......48 years ago. We were married on January 13, 1968. God knew that this young man would be the one who would be with me in sickness and in health.....for better, for worse, for richer, for poorer...to love and to cherish me 'till death do us part. We have certainly had our share of good times and bad times.....sickness and health.... joy and pain.... sunshine as well as rain....and we've been through "thick and thin" and many "trials and tribulations".............. but my husband is the **one and only one** for **me!**

God knew this would be the one who I would need beside me in 1987 during my battle against cancer and He knew this would be the one and only one who could help me write this book and deliver this message of hope to you. He was by my side through it all. He preserved all of the medical records, files and reports in chronological order. So he knows every detail of this story from the diagnosis to the victory and beyond.

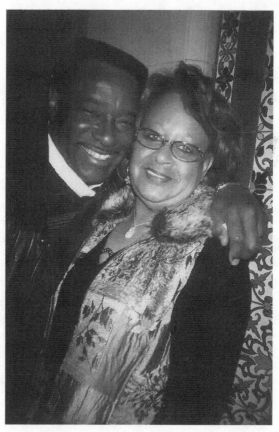

On August 15, 1968, we were blessed with our son, Melvin Jr.

Baby Melvin

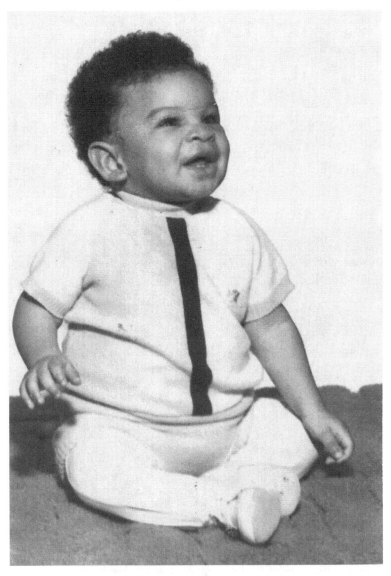

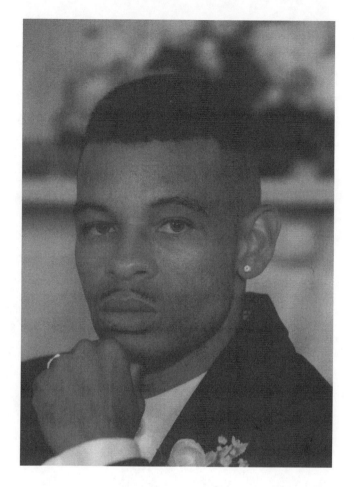

## All Grown Up

God plants many "seeds of greatness" in every child He creates. On August 31, 1990, twenty two years after creating Melvin, Jr., He used one of those "seeds of greatness" to create Melvin, III. That's just one of the reasons He created Melvin, Jr. in the first place. It's easy to see why everybody in the "generational line" is so special and so important to the next generation. You never know what God is going to do next. He could use one of your "seeds of greatness" to bring forth the child who will grow up and become the Scientist, the Doctor or the Research Specialist who will develop the cure for cancer. God already has the cure. It's just a matter of Him choosing the person He wants to work through to bring forth those formulas and the cure. Hopefully, that person has already been created and is on the verge of a **DIVINE** revelation that will lead to the cure for this dreaded disease.

On August 31, 1990, we were blessed with our grandson,
Melvin III.

Melvin Pierre, III (Baby Photo)

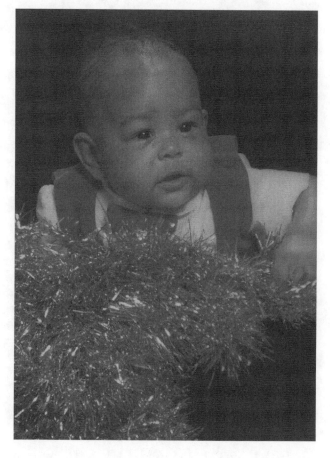

Melvin Pierre, III @ 18 Years of Age

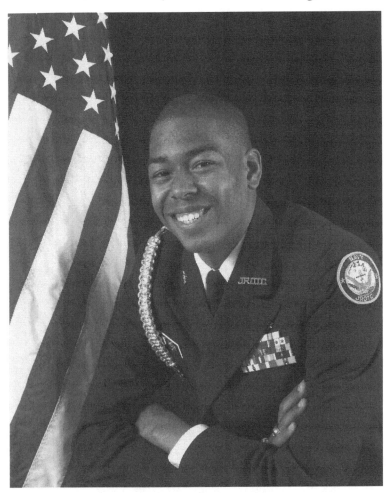

On August 31, 2011, Melvin, III will marked his 21st birthday. He's currently completing the requirements for his college degree. His goal is to start his career as a 2nd Lieutenant in the United States Air Force. He will be the 1st Pierre to reach that level of success. We are all looking forward to his graduation and to him earning the commission to begin his career.

I know most of you have a fantastic relationship with your family. I know you feel the same way about your family as I do mine. But I was having a conversation with a young lady, a few days before Mother's Day, 2011, and what she shared with me took my breath away. She stated she had not **spoken** to her Mother for over two years. That's her choice. However, from my perspective, that's unfortunate. After 64 years of living, I can tell you this for sure:

## Grandma & Grandpa, Momma & Daddy, Brothers & Sisters, Sons & Daughters, Grandsons and Granddaughters, Uncles and Aunts

## Are Here For A *Limited Time Only* & Are *Irreplaceable!!!*

# Shower Them With Your Love... Right Here & Now

This is the one and only time we have to spend together. When the "appointed time" has come for a family member to leave and "cross back over," they won't be coming back. When **you** leave, **you** won't be coming back. Make sure you have every family member on a DVD so you'll always have an audio and video record of their beautiful smiles because tomorrow is promised to no one. To the young lady who hasn't communicated with her mother in over two years, and to any others who may be in the same situation with your parents, grandparents, brothers, sisters, sons and daughters, grandsons and granddaughters, uncles and aunts, I would like to share the following: This is **your** moment and **their** moment. This is **your** time and **their** time. We are here **NOW**. We hope to be here tomorrow.....but we have not arrived at that destination yet. **NOW** is the time. This is our one and only window of opportunity to enjoy each other.... grow "young" or old together...... and to just share our lives together.

After you finish reading this page, may I suggest that you call Momma, Daddy, Grandma and Grandpa just to say **THANKS** for being there for all of **your** years when you **really** needed them.....**THANKS** for being there to guide you when you couldn't guide yourself.....**THANKS** for sharing their wisdom and vision with you.....**THANKS** for all of the sacrifices they made in order for you to have a better life.

Take time out of your busy schedule to share breakfast, lunch or dinner with and ask :

> **"What can I do to help make your life better?"**

> **"Is there any place you have not been that you'd like to go?"**

> **"Is there anything you haven't done that you'd like to do?"**

**Listen** very carefully to their answers and start making plans to turn their dreams into reality. **NOW** is the time! My mom always wanted to go to Las Vegas. My husband and I took her to Las Vegas and she had so much fun, she talked about that trip until the end of "her" time. Those are the kind of memories that can live on as long as you live ....priceless moments that you want to cherish. If your parents or grandparents have never been on an airplane......take them to whatever destination their hearts desire.....and watch the tears in their eyes as their dreams unfold right in front of them. This is important because our parents and/or grandparents made our dreams come true when we were kids and now the tables are "turned.' So why not make some of their dreams come true? **NOW** is the time!

Some of us have a tendency to spend more time with our "friends" than our family. Over the years, many "friends" have come and gone....but there is nothing in this world like your **family**.

At the end of the day, nobody cares about you like your **family**. And remember: this is the family that God chose to put you in. You didn't put yourself in this family. On your date of birth, you opened up your eyes....came to life and all of these big people were smiling at you. They were glad you had arrived. And they will be sorry to see you leave. While you are here, there will be ups and downs.....drama here.....drama there...and drama everywhere....but they are still your family members and nobody can ever replace any of them. Your sisters and brothers can never be replaced. Your kids and grandkids can never be replaced. Your Mother and Father can never be replaced. These are the two people that God chose to bring you here. Were it not for those exact two people, where would you be?

I hope and pray you have a great relationship with your Mother and Father because we only have one life to live.....one chance to share and spend our lives together. If you are in a situation where the relationships are not right, I would encourage you to do whatever needs to be done to make those relationships right. Maybe you're still mad because of a "spanking" you got when you were young and mischievous. Maybe you're still mad because you feel like your parents showed favoritism to one of your brothers or sisters. Maybe you're still mad at your Momma or your Daddy because they didn't approve of your first "love." Maybe you're still mad because they were too strict on you. Maybe you're still mad at your older brother or sister who had to "discipline" you when your Mom and Dad were not home. Maybe you're still mad at your little sister or brother because they broke one of your favorite toys. Whatever it is......**<u>FIX IT NOW</u>**.....**<u>MAKE IT RIGHT</u>**....because time waits for no one. Start the relationship all over again.......because.....in an instant, any one of them (or you) could be gone. It's worth it to fix it now and make it right.

Here's a very personal story that I'll share with you. My husband's mother and father separated and divorced when he was about 5 years old. He can't ever remember living in a household with his father. His father, who was an Army veteran, was transferred to the state of Washington and then on to California. The relationship was never right. There never was an "emotional connection" between father and son. His father passed away in 1982 and the "lack of a father-son relationship" still troubles him to this day. A few years ago, he reached a point where he could use the words "my daddy" because he realized had it not been for his daddy, he would not be here today. As a child, he was focused on what his daddy had **not** done for him....but missed what his daddy had **REALLY DONE** for him **to even be here**.....**alive and breathing in 2011**. He'll never get another opportunity to make that relationship right. But you have an opportunity, right now, to make **yours** right.

As I said, if you are in a situation where you are "hostile, alienated or otherwise estranged" from your parents, grandparents, brothers or sisters, sons and daughters, grandsons or granddaughters or other loved ones.....**<u>FIX IT NOW. MAKE IT RIGHT!!</u>**

**NOW** is the time........because you don't want to find yourself in a situation where their time has expired and you're standing there crying and saying to yourself... "if I coulda-woulda-shoulda".........but they can't hear you no more.

I would encourage you to visit YOU TUBE © and watch **James Taylor** "Live" as he delivers the message in his song

**<u>"Shower The People You Love With Love...Show Them The Way That You Feel©"</u>**

Here's the link to the "Live" performance:

**<u>Shower The People Copy this link into your browser © by James Taylor</u>**

<u>http://www.youtube.com/watch?v=tydSHv9ak8E&feature=related</u>

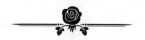

# 30,000 Days To Live- A New Perspective On Life

When you go through a challenging medical condition and survive it, you realize there are things in life that **are important**....and then there are things in life that are **not so important**. You realize that you are a mortal human being with a date of birth (sunrise) and an upcoming date of "death" (sunset). No matter how much money you may have or may not have, there **will be** a sunset....an "expiration date." The average life expectancy, per the "experts," for a female in America, is somewhere around 79.5 years. That's about 29,000+ days to live. I just made my 64th birthday. So I've already lived 23,360 days of my life expectancy.....8,760 after my cancer diagnosis.

In our family, my dad lived 67 years (approximately 24,455 days). My mom lived 95 years (approximately 34,675 days). My grandfather lived to 100 (approximately 36,500 days). It's mind-boggling to think that God has blessed me with 23,360 days thus far. How many days has He blessed you with so far?

We don't know what the future holds....but we know **Who** holds the future.

**I BELIEVE** , when we reach the last day of life (as we know it), God closes our "window of life" at the same time He activates the "white light of peace and serenity" so our spirit can find its way safely home and back in HIS arms.

**God, Our Creator** is the **One & Only One** who is in control.

He's the One who wakes us up in the morning and gives us the opportunity to live another day. Nobody has a lease on life! Some folks who are here today will not be here tomorrow...and some folks who are not here today will be born tomorrow. You may or may not have heard this before.....but I'll say it again:

**YESTERDAY** has come and gone......**TOMORROW**...we may never see. That's why we call **TODAY**.....the **"PRESENT."** Because that's exactly what it is..............**a Present**...........
**the Present........ A Direct Gift from GOD.**

Every second...every moment....every hour.....every day is a direct gift from our **Creator.** It's a **PRESENT.** So let's cherish it as if it's our last one.....because it very well could be. Let's concentrate on what's going right in our life....instead of what's going wrong. That's what I had to do to make it through.

We all look at life through a different set of lenses. We all have a different point of view. I learned a long time ago that **YOUR PERCEPTION** is **YOUR REALITY**.

**You** see what **You** see and **You** believe what **You** believe. I'm not trying to change anything you believe. We're all free to believe whatever we want to believe. One person will see it one way and another person will look at the exact same thing and come to a very different conclusion. That's normal. That's human. However, before I close this chapter, I'd like to share some "food for thought" with you:

# I BELIEVE

Every human being God creates is made with a special purpose. God don't make no junk!! As we go through life, it's up to us to discover that purpose. Once we discover that purpose, we'll be in a "position" to fulfill the purpose He had in mind when he created us. Every **BODY** (and I do mean every human body) He creates is a work of art.....an absolute masterpiece..... handcrafted by the Creator.

\*\*\*\*\*\*\*\*\*\*\*\*\*\*\*\*\*\*\*\*\*\*\*\*\*\*\*\*\*\*\*\*\*\*\*\*\*\*\*\*\*\*\*\*\*\*\*\*

Take a look at this excerpt that was posted on the internet by Mike Collett-White / Reuters- Tuesday, June 28, 2011 ©.

## Francis Bacon work fetches $29 million at auction

REUTERS *By Mike Collett-White | Reuters – Tue, Jun 28, 2011*

LONDON (Reuters Life!) - A painting by Irish-born artist Francis Bacon sold for 18.0 million pounds ($28.7 million) on Tuesday, the second highest price paid for a work of art at a Christie's post-war and contemporary auction in London.

"Study for a Portrait," depicting a besuited man seated on a gilded armchair enshrouded in a sea of blue, had been expected to fetch around 11 million pounds, although the sale price includes a buyer's premium which the estimate does not.

\*\*\*\*\*\*\*\*\*\*\*\*\*\*\*\*\*\*\*\*\*\*\*\*\*\*\*\*\*\*\*\*\*\*\*\*\*\*\*\*\*\*\*\*\*\*\*\*

If "one painting", created by a "human being" that God created, is worth $28.7 million dollars, then what's the "value" of **one human being** who is created on God's canvas worth? Each one of us is a one of a kind, hand-molded, hand crafted, personally painted, certified "portrait" created by God. We are all **authenticated** originals and can never be duplicated. There has never been and never will be another **YOU!** So you are very, very special......no matter what others say or think about you. **Their** opinions don't matter because they are a human being just like you.

## Don't Ever Let Another Human Being Put You Down

*Nobody knows how great you are....or how great you can be....except HE who made you. Don't ever let another human being make you feel like you're inferior to them.....because you're not!!*

YOU ARE JUST AS IMPORTANT TO **GOD** AS ANY OF HIS OTHER CHILDREN ARE!

We all have the right and a free will to believe whatever we want to believe and, as I stated in the very beginning of this book, I'm not trying to impose my beliefs on you about anything. Just want to share some things to "think" about.

Over the years, I've heard some people (not many) say they'll believe it when they "see" it. "They" say they want to see God perform miracles in modern times **before** they'll believe in Him.

They'll believe when they "see." That's their choice. They "see" miracles everyday…and still don't "see." To them, the records in the Bible or what He has done in the past are not relevant today. The truth of the matter is that the Creator does not have to prove anything to anybody for any reason…..especially to those He created. But here's a "modern-day miracle" we "see" every day and one that every generation has seen for all of their days:

# Childbirth Is A Miracle All By Itself

I submit to you that 365 days a year, in every country, a child is born. A child is a direct gift from God. That's a miracle all by itself. **Who** else can combine sperm and an egg or several eggs and create a human being or duplicates, triplicates, or even quadruplets…..most with 10 fingers…10 toes…2 ears…2 eyes…2 arms… 2 legs…hair in all the right places…with beautiful, "heal-able" skin…complete with an immune system…a neurological system where every cell of the body has a nerve component…a reproductive system that's activated at the proper time… a cardio-vascular system…a gastro-intestinal system…a once in a lifetime, one of a kind voice…a comprehensive bone structure to support all of that…and many other parts, systems and processes that I can't began to name or understand…and then He tops it off with the most awesome **Central Processing System** known to man…..the **human brain**, which, in some cases, can retain 100 years of memories!!! **Who** else has that kind of power??? It's amazing to watch God work as we leave His hands and open up our eyes in our Mother's arms. At the end of our term in the "oven," He opens up the "window of life"……turns on the spotlight and introduces us to the world as one of His newest creations. And He stays connected to every human being He creates…from the beginning to the end. The human being might not want to stay connected…but He's always there for us. His network spans the universe and beyond.

You can believe it or not believe it. That's up to you. That's a choice you have to make…..one way or the other. As for me and my house, **WE BELIEVE!!!**

In my opinion, childbirth is one of the greatest miracles you'll ever witness. All the hearts He creates are the same color and work exactly the same. All kidneys are the same color and work exactly the same. All lungs are the same color and work exactly the same. There are times when a tragedy may strike one family but could change the future outlook for several other families at the same time….because some families, in all of their grief, may be generous enough to donate the heart, lungs, kidneys, and other internal organs of their loved ones to others and, if there's a match, those internal organs can continue to work in the recipient of those organs. The donor could be from one country and culture and the recipient could be from a totally different country and culture. The hearts, lungs, kidneys and other vital organs have no interest in the race, the color, economic status, language, culture or religious affiliation of the donor or the recipient. If there's a "match," the organs of the donor could improve the quality of life for the recipient. For example, a billionaire and a pauper have the same internal "operating" systems and organs…. with red blood running through their veins. There's no such thing as "blue" blood as some people claim to have. If the billionaire needed a heart, lung, kidney or liver transplant and the pauper was a "perfect match," the billionaire would gladly accept the organs of the pauper without ever asking about the color of the pauper's skin. And **Who** has to give **His Blessings** in order for those organs to continue to work?  The Creator!!!

A Rolls-Royce is a Rolls-Royce; a Ferrari is a Ferrari; a Bentley is a Bentley; a Maserati is a Maserati; a Cadillac is a Cadillac; a Human Being is a Human Being. Is the Madeira Red Rolls-Royce better than the Metropolitan Blue Rolls-Royce? Is the Yellow Maserati better than the Victory Blue Maserati? Is the Black Bentley better than the Silver Tempest Bentley? Is the brown Human Being better than the pink Human Being? Or is the beige Human Being better than the brown Human Being? Is one better than the other? **Absolutely not!!!** Just like you can't judge a book by its "cover"........ you can't judge a human being by the "cover." We've got to look for the "**beauty and the character beyond the cover.**" Not only should we "reach across the racial, cultural, economic and other imaginary aisles and lines" to better understand one another and the gifts God gave each one of us to help each other.......we should "reach across the continents" and look for the "**beauty and the character beyond the cover**"as well. By doing so, we can start the process of tearing down the walls of **animosity and distrust** and start building **a spirit of cooperation and understanding.**

The world has its own color-coding system that is used to "define" human beings when, in fact, we have absolutely nothing to do with the skin tones God chooses for each one of us to be. God knows exactly what He's doing. We don't.....but He does! The skin tone that God decides to paint us with does not make one better or worse than the other......successful or unsuccessful....a good person or a menace to society.....a prince or a pauper.....a caring person or a non-caring person.....a giver or a taker..... or a person who is entitled to anything! When He creates us, He gives us his **blessing** and starts us off with a clean heart, a clean mind, a clean slate, seeds of greatness, special talents, the gift of time, a roadmap and a set of "holy scriptures and laws" written in the Bible over 2,000 years ago and the "freedom" to make whatever choices we want to make. Then we start this journey called **LIFE** and start making choices as we develop our character, aptitudes, attitudes and other learned behaviors. The **choices** we make will determine our **destiny.**

It doesn't matter what country or continent we come from because, if the truth be told, we are much more alike than we are different. **I BELIEVE** that **every** human being God creates is important to Him. When we criticize what He creates, we are criticizing Him. We may not want to admit it or acknowledge it or even acknowledge Him, but we are all brothers and sisters... because we all come from the same Creator. In His eyes, no human being is more important than the other. We are all His children.......children that He has personally created. It is mind-boggling to think that God is the Creator of **every human being**.....past, present and future....on every continent on this planet! He is **Omnipotent** and **Omnipresent** and can oversee and bless the birth of every child everywhere all at once........ in addition to taking care of all of our needs, answering all of our prayers, and attending to every other detail in His universe!! What an awesome God!!! If you want to see a Picasso, a Rembrandt, or a Frances Bacon work of art, I'm sure you can find a picture of many of those on the internet. On the other hand, if you want to see a "walking, talking, breathing, talented "work of art" that God created, just look in the mirror. When you look in the mirror, what you'll see is God's gift to **you**!!!

## YOU ARE A MIRACLE BECAUSE GOD CREATED YOU!

But the question is "What will our gift back to Him be..... after being here for 10,000-20,000-30,000 days or whatever time He has allotted to us? He plants "seeds of greatness" in every one of us. When we come to the end of our road and have an opportunity to review the DVD of our lives with Him, will He be pleased? Will **you** be pleased? Dr. Martin Luther King, Jr. had a dream that, one day (and I hope I live to see that day), we would live in a nation where we will not be judged by the color of our skin…but by the content of our character. God **will not be** impressed by the color (cover) of the skin that He gave us…. but He will be impressed by the <u>**content of the character…..**</u> <u>**beyond the cover He gave us.**</u> That's the part we develop and have control over.

His doors are open 24 hours a day… every day. And He's **always** home…..and ready to listen to each and every one of us. I found out, for myself, that if we take the time to pray, He'll take the time to answer our prayers. If **we will**…….**He will.**

### <u>Enjoy Your Life…..TIME Is A Very</u> <u>Special & Precious Gift!!!</u>

Don't ever be too "proud" to get down on your knees and ask God for His Guidance.  We are not here **by accident.** We are here <u>**on purpose**</u>….<u>**for**</u> a purpose…at <u>**this**</u> time. We didn't just randomly appear out of nowhere. We were created for a very special reason. If we **seek** it, we will **find** it.  As for me and my house, we will continue to serve the Lord and find joy in every second, every moment, every hour and every day that we have left on this earth. We intend to spread as much joy and sunshine to others as we can. We intend to **LIVE** every day to **the fullest!!!** We intend to look for the "**beauty and the character beyond the cover**" in every individual we encounter. We will do our very best to follow the Golden Rule:

"Do unto others as you would
have them do unto you"

# What About YOU?

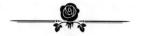

# Lagniappe "A Little Something Extra"

In Louisiana, we always try to give "a little something extra." That's what we call **Lagniappe.** If you go to a bakery in Louisiana and buy a dozen of donuts and, to your surprise, find 13 in the bag......that extra one is called **Lagniappe.** If you order 12 Hot Wings in a restaurant and you find 13, that's **Lagniappe.** This special message for young folks is **Lagniappe- A Little Something Extra.**

## A SPECIAL MESSAGE FOR YOUNG FOLKS

There are **good** forces and **bad** forces in this world. Beware of the "spiritual" warfare that's going on all around you...every day. It's for real. The minute you reach the point in your life when you "think" you can think for yourself, satan will attack you and your "mental" computer....your mind....the central processing unit God created. Every "new creation" is created with a "blank disk" on their mental computer. The programs and the "software" that are added to your "mental" computer, as you live life, will determine your destiny. If you don't choose God and seek His guidance...Satan will automatically choose you and guide you into a web of deception and corrupt the files in your head. He wants you to join his congregation and become one of his disciples. His mission is to destroy your heart, mind, body, soul, spirit as well as your dignity! His goal is to put a "virus" on your central processing unit….and destroy all the "do-whats-right files" on your brain. Trying to go through life without a relationship with your Creator is like operating your computer without anti-virus protection and firewall protection. You **will** get hacked! The HACKER (satan-the devil-the serpent-the "snake in the grass" or whatever you want to call him) will corrupt the system that controls all of your thought processes. Before you know it, he will "hack" into your system and take control of your brain and your life, **remotely,** with all kinds of temptations, deceptions, vices and devices, schemes, scams, smoke and mirrors, and mind-altering substances that may "appear to be cool" and make you feel good (**temporarily**) …..but will cause you to get hooked and dependent on those substances to the point where you'll have to keep coming back for more and more and more. Once that happens, he'll have complete control of your mind and your time. **"Everything that glitters ain't gold!"** You are no match for satan….by yourself.

He has mastered the techniques of working through a "select group or gang" of your peers to recruit you and lead you down a path of destruction and corruption that will cause you to waste many valuable years before you can find your way back to the "table of blessings" that God has prepared and have in store for you. Stay close to your parents… for they have a wealth of knowledge, wisdom and experience. In your own family, you probably have family members in every age bracket….. 5-10-15-20-30-40-50-60-70 and 80. Don't seek advice from those who are the same age as you….because their knowledge is limited just like yours. On the contrary, seek advice from those who have already passed the "mile-markers" that you hope to pass some day. They can tell you what to expect before you get there. Pay attention and learn from them. They want the best for you. Honor your Father and Mother at all times. God sent them here **before you arrived**........so they could be "Lamplighters" and "Guiding Lights" for **your** life. There is no way you can know what they know because you haven't been here long enough. There is no way you can have enough vision to see what they've already seen. You don't have to believe me or my words. Pick up a B-I-B-L-E and read it for yourself and find out how satan deceived the first man (Adam) and the first women (Eve) in the Garden of Eden. The B-I-B-L-E is the Word of God and the "instruction manual" that was created for human beings. I've heard folks say...and I agree... that the **B-I-B-L-E** will provide you with some **B**asic-**I**nstructions-**B**efore-**L**eaving-**E**arth! Get informed and be prepared as you work your way through Life. Follow the One who created you so you can find your purpose in Life. You'll be glad you did.

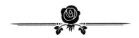

# Closing Remarks

If you or any of your family members are fighting this dreaded disease right now, surround yourself and your family with as many **positive people** as you can. **Eliminate** all of the "**toxic**" people, in your life, *immediately,* because one "toxic" person can take all of the wind out of your sails and keep you focused on "the gloom and the doom." They can drain all of the "sunshine" out of a room, out of your heart and out of your spirit…. just by walking in the room. Their negative thoughts, words and actions will keep you in a constant state of depression and create an atmosphere of **doubt** in your conscious and subconscious mind as well as in your spirit. You cannot achieve a **positive** outcome if you are in a constant state of depression and doubt. When I was diagnosed in 1987 and was forced into the "fight of my life," I never gave any consideration whatsoever to dying during **that** particular fight. I found out that **"Things turn out best for those who make the best out of the way things turn out!"** Expect the best. Expect positive results.

### You Can't Fight Cancer If You Don't Have Hope!!!!

**Hope** is what you need to make it from day to day. **Hope** is what you need to give yourself a "fighting chance" to win the battle. If you don't have **Hope,** you'll give up and give in without a fight…..without ever knowing what would have been possible. As long as there's warm blood running in your veins, **Don't Give Up**………and **Don't Give In**….because you still have **time to pray.** Hold your head up high and fight with all the strength you can muster………because, no matter what the "report" says, it ain't over until God says it's over. Folks can say whatever they want to say and predict whatever they want to predict……but it ain't over until God says it is finished and certifies that your time has expired. With God on your side, **anything** can happen at **any time.** With God………… **All Things Are Possible!!!**

As I look back on my 64 years, I've had my share of ups and downs and turnarounds. But by the grace of God, I've been here over 23,360 days thus far. That's a lot of days. Has it been worth it? In spite of all that I've been through, I can assure you that my good days still outweigh my bad days by an astronomical margin. After 95 years of living, my momma felt the same way.

<u>"**I Won't Complain**©"</u> was one of her favorite songs.

If you have access to a computer, I would encourage you to go to YOU TUBE© and listen to one of our favorite gospel singers, **<u>Theorlyn Rayborn,</u>** from Lake Charles, Louisiana as she offers her rendition of <u>"**I Won't Complain** ©."</u>

Here's the link:

**<u>Theorlyn Rayborn</u>**

**<u>I Won't Complain©</u>**

<u>http://www.youtube.com/watch?v=TcTwbpPdgf0</u>

Please continue to **Support Cancer Research** and all of the organizations and support groups that are engaged in the battle against this dreaded disease. I would also ask you to seek out and consider helping someone in your own home town who may be facing a battle against cancer. They would appreciate it if you would volunteer to help in any way you can.

- Accompany them to a chemotherapy session and give their family a break.

- Volunteer to sit with them at home or at the hospital to give their family members an opportunity to enjoy some quality time away from the situation.

- Take them for a "walk and a talk."

- Or maybe a drive by the lake or a day at the beach.

- Treat them to breakfast, lunch or dinner at one of their favorite restaurants.

- **Let them talk**.... **while you listen**.... as they share some of the good times they've enjoyed in their life.

- Maintain their lawn and garden.

- Make sure their kids get to and from school and to and from other appointments safely.

- Help with the cleaning so they won't have to worry about that.

- Help them to find their joy....in the middle of their storm.

- Give them some space and help them to find peace and an opportunity to enjoy a good night's sleep. Let them call you at 11:00am. when **they** wake up instead of you calling them at 7:00am when <u>you</u> wake up. Under the circumstances, their night may not have been as peaceful as yours.

- If you are in a financial position to do so, **accompany** them to the hospital's business office or to one of their doctor's offices and pay $100 or whatever you can afford to pay on one of their medical bills to help relieve some of those financial burdens. They'll probably never ask you to do that. So just ask them if you can help them in that way.

- Or simply ask them what you can do to help make their lives better during this difficult time.

What they need is for someone to come along and put a smile in their heart. I was surrounded by all of my family members and so many beautiful people who brought "**sunshine**" when they came to see me. It helped to keep my mind off of Biopsies, Surgeries, Radiation, Chemotherapy, PET Scans, CT Scans, X-Rays, Blood Profiles, Tamoxifen and all of the other things I was going through. What I needed and what your friends, who are battling this disease, need is a daily dose of "**sunshine**." I'm sure you can find a way to provide that. So I'm asking <u>**YOU**</u> to bring some "**sunshine**" to somebody's house and put a smile in somebody's heart...today....tomorrow...the next day.....and the next day.

# A Simple Prayer

Lord, make me an instrument of your peace.

Where there is hatred...let me sow love.

Where there is injury...pardon.

Where there is doubt...faith.

Where there is despair...hope.

Where there is darkness...light.

Where there is sadness...joy.

O Divine Master, grant that I may

not so much seek

To be consoled...as to console,

To be understood...as to understand,

To be loved...as to love,

For

It is in giving...that we receive,

It is in pardoning...that we are pardoned,

It is in dying...that we are born
to eternal life.

Saint Francis

As you continue your journey down the highway of life, there will be road blocks, detours, construction as well as destruction. I pray that **GOD WILL CONTINUE TO GUIDE YOU AND BLESS EVERY STEP YOU TAKE!!!**

### <u>Peace & Many Blessings For You & Every Member Of Your Family</u>

Patricia Ann Penn Pierre

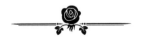

# About The Author

Patricia Ann Penn Pierre was born and raised in New Orleans, Louisiana. She is the sixth child of Samuel & Beatrice Penn. In August, 1987, her life changed, dramatically, when she was diagnosed with breast cancer and was faced with having to have a double mastectomy. She made a decision, early on in the process, to turn it all over to <u>GOD</u> and let <u>HIM</u> lead her through the valley of the shadow of death. She had never been to a place this dark before....so she had no choice but to <u>Walk By Faith</u> because there was no sight! At first glance, the odds may have been stacked against her, but <u>GOD</u> turned everything around in her favor. This is an incredible story of <u>Faith, Hope, Love & Courage.</u> In the face of adversity, her FAITH never wavered. This period in her life is the "defining moment" when <u>GOD</u> and <u>HIS WORD</u> came alive in her life. This is her story...her <u>Message of Hope</u> for you..... that no matter what the situation may be, or appear to be, <u>GOD</u> is in control and <u>GOD ANSWERS PRAYERS.</u> You are invited to "step back in time" as she recounts her "journey through the valley," and her ultimate <u>VICTORY</u> over cancer.

She has shared her story with folks all across America and in places as far away as Barbados. Each time she has shared this powerful testimony, folks have surrounded her to share the fact that they were encouraged to "keep their hopes up high and to keep pressing forward........ with great expectations" in their fight against this dreaded disease. In the midst of her storm, her <u>FAITH</u> increased ten-fold and she was able to focus on what she was going <u>TO</u> ( Victory ) instead of what she was going <u>THROUGH</u> (surgeries and chemotherapy). This is truly <u>A Message of Hope</u>.......from a 24 Year Cancer Survivor.

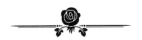

# EMERGENCY NUMBERS

### Call J-E-S-U-S.

He Will Answer Your Call.

Available 24 Hours A Day-Every Day-Holidays, Nights and
Weekends Included.

No Telephone or Internet Service Need.

Operator Assistance Is Not Necessary.

Direct Connections.
No Fancy Voice Mail System To Navigate.

No Busy Signals.

If you feel lonely, in danger, in trouble, down and out,
depressed,  worried, need help, guidance or you just want
to THANK HIM or PRAISE HIM, call J-E-S-U-S.
He's awaiting your call.

Here's what the Bible says about Jesus Christ in John 10-30:

"I and my Father are one."

# YOUR <u>SFGTD</u> BOX ©

If you have access to a computer, please go to YOU TUBE © and receive the information on the **SFGTD** Box ©. This is your **SOMETHING FOR GOD TO DO** Box. © Put your prayer requests in writing and place them in your **SFGTD** Box © and watch God work on your behalf.

Copy this link into your browser:

http://www.youtube.com/watch?v=6zaQmzRABzg

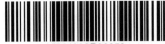
10564099R00059

Made in the USA
Charleston, SC
14 December 2011